Ana Almeida Ribeiro
Nuno Ferreira
Paula Flores

Pedagogical Manual

Ana Almeida Ribeiro
Nuno Ferreira
Paula Flores

Pedagogical Manual

Therapeutic Management and Administration

ScienciaScripts

Imprint

Cover image: www.ingimage.com

This book is a translation from the original published under ISBN 978-620-6-76011-5.

Publisher:
Sciencia Scripts
is a trademark of
Dodo Books Indian Ocean Ltd. and OmniScriptum S.R.L publishing group

120 High Road, East Finchley, London, N2 9ED, United Kingdom
Str. Armeneasca 28/1, office 1, Chisinau MD-2012, Republic of Moldova, Europe
Printed at: see last page
ISBN: 978-620-7-65995-1

Those who confess their mistakes are wiser today than they were yesterday.
Alexander Pope

Index

Introduction:

The nursing profession requires a combination of technical competence, scientific knowledge and interpersonal skills. This teaching manual has been developed with the aim of providing nursing students with a comprehensive resource that addresses all of these aspects through the lens of drug administration and therapeutic management. Each section of the manual has been meticulously structured to ensure that students can navigate the complex procedures of medication administration with confidence and care. Throughout the manual, we emphasise the importance of understanding pharmacology, pharmacokinetics and pharmacodynamics as the foundations for effective drug administration. In addition, the need to understand the various routes of administration, the risks associated with each, and specific techniques to minimise complications are discussed in detail. This knowledge is vital to ensure that medicines contribute to the patient's recovery and well-being, while minimising the risks of adverse effects.

The manual also addresses the importance of communication in nursing practice, an essential skill for any nurse who interacts not only with patients, but also with family members and other healthcare professionals. The ability to effectively communicate the care plan, explain procedures and listen to patients' concerns is fundamental to therapeutic success and patient satisfaction.

This manual not only serves as an introduction to basic nursing procedures, but also as a quick reference guide for everyday situations in the hospital, promoting patient safety and effective healthcare.

With this resource, we hope to equip future nurses with the tools they need to act with confidence and precision, raising the standard of care provided and contributing to safer, evidence-based nursing practice.

Chapter 1: Promotion and Management of the Therapeutic Regimen

The management and promotion of the therapeutic regime are fundamental aspects of nursing practice, involving the correct administration of medicines and close monitoring of the patient. This chapter aims to introduce nursing students to key concepts and essential practices to ensure the safe and effective administration of medicines.

1.1 Basic Principles of Drug Administration

Background and importance

Medication administration is a critical component of nursing practice that requires rigour and precision to ensure both the safety and therapeutic efficacy of the treatment. This process involves several fundamental stages, from the medical prescription to the delivery and monitoring of the medication to the patient (Amendoeira, 2006).

The challenge of adhering to the therapeutic regime

In everyday life, despite the wide dissemination of information, many individuals persist in adopting inappropriate lifestyle habits or do not adhere to prescribed therapeutic regimes, jeopardising their health and quality of life. This discrepancy between knowledge and action can be attributed to multiple factors, including the complexity of therapeutic regimes and a lack of understanding of the consequences of non-adherence (Amendoeira, 2006).

Lack of adherence not only reduces the effectiveness of treatments, but also imposes significant costs on health systems due to increased complications and the need for additional treatments, posing a substantial challenge in the management of chronic diseases (Kérouac et al., 1996).

Education for Self-Management

To improve adherence to the therapeutic regime, self-management education is essential. Teaching patients and carers how to manage their treatment effectively, providing them with the knowledge and tools to make informed decisions, is a proven effective strategy

(Kérouac et al., 1996). This education should include detailed information about the disease, the drugs prescribed, their actions, potential side effects and the critical importance of maintaining the prescribed therapeutic regime.

The role of the health professional

Success in promoting an effective therapeutic regime depends heavily on the healthcare professional responsible for its implementation. Nurses play a vital role, not only in the direct administration of medication, but also in the educational and emotional support of patients (Amendoeira, 2006). Nurses value the patient's active role in their treatment, establishing an interpersonal relationship that allows for a more personalised approach geared towards therapeutic success.

Integrating Virginia Henderson's principles into nursing practice can broaden this approach, promoting care that respects the dignity and autonomy of the patient, focusing not only on the physical aspects of treatment, but also on their emotional, social and spiritual needs (Raharja et al., 2022).

Medicines administration is a complex area of practice that requires in-depth knowledge from healthcare professionals, sharp practical skills and a patient-centred approach. Effective education and management strategies, the use of technology and the application of holistic care principles are essential to ensure treatment effectiveness and patient safety (Raharja et al., 2022).

1.2 Prevention of Medication Errors

The prevention of errors in the administration of medicines is a central concern in patient safety and requires a multidimensional and integrated approach, as advocated by Virginia Henderson's principles. The emphasis on individualised, patient-centred care is fundamental to improving the safety and effectiveness of healthcare.

Adoption of Virginia Henderson's principles

Virginia Henderson's principles highlight the importance of considering the individual as a whole, emphasising personalised care in all interactions with the patient. This approach not only helps to establish a relationship of trust and mutual respect between the nurse and the patient, but also increases the ability of both to effectively manage the therapeutic regime. (2023), the continuous training of nurses is vital to ensure that they have the necessary skills to apply these principles in their daily lives, thus reducing the likelihood of errors.

Technology and Continuing Education

Technology plays a crucial role in minimising medication errors. Computerised prescription systems, for example, help to eliminate transcription errors and ensure that prescriptions are clear and precise. Similarly, barcode scanning during medication administration ensures that the right medication is administered in the right dose, to the right patient and at the right time. These technological tools, combined with continuous training, are essential for keeping nurses up to date with best practices and new technologies, as advocated by Siboni et al (2023).

Safety barriers and near *miss* identification

According to the risk management model, inspired by Reason's "Swiss Cheese Model", healthcare organisations must implement multiple security barriers to prevent errors. Each layer of protection can intercept a potential error, preventing it from reaching the patient. Identifying *near misses*, which are incidents that did not cause harm to the patient but had the potential to do so, is also crucial. Analysing and learning from these near misses allows preventive measures to be implemented before real harm occurs.

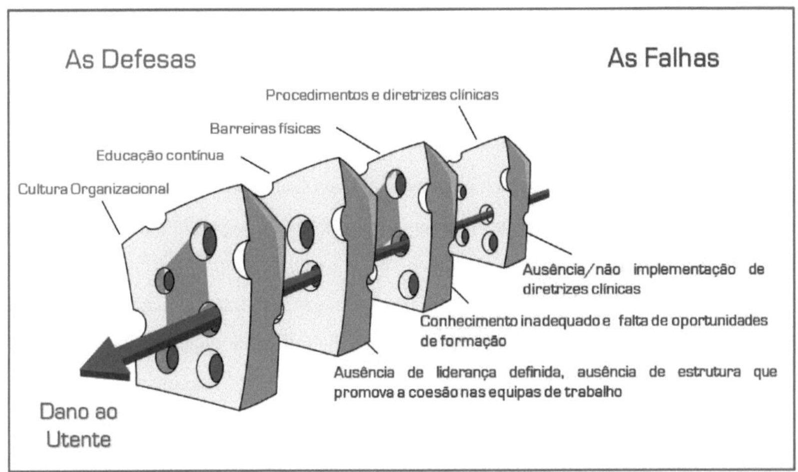

Swiss cheese model, adapted from James Reason, 2000

Promoting a culture of safety

It is essential to promote a safety culture in which errors are seen as opportunities for learning and improvement. This culture encourages open reporting and discussion of errors and near misses, without penalties, with a focus on continuous process improvement. Integrating Virginia Henderson's principles into this safety culture ensures that patient care is always personalised and focused on their specific needs, helping to prevent errors by promoting safer and more effective practices.

Preventing errors in drug administration and the importance of the "right nine"

When discussing the fundamentals of drug administration, it is crucial to consider the evolution of traditional concepts towards a more comprehensive and precise approach. Previously, practice emphasised the "right five" of drug administration, which included the right patient, the right drug, the right dose, the right route and the right time. However, with the advancement of patient safety, new elements have been incorporated, resulting in the "nine rights" of drug administration (Pinheiro et al., 2021; Carvalho et al., 2021).

The "nine rights" of medication administration cover not only the traditional aspects, but also consider the right expiry date, the right approach, the right time, the right forecast, the right record, the right action, the right form, the right response and drug compatibility. This more comprehensive approach aims to ensure patient safety, reduce medication errors and promote quality care (Carvalho et al., 2021). The preparation and administration of medicines requires attention to detail and adherence to established protocols.

Constant supervision of the nursing team, together with their contribution to drawing up and adapting protocols, is essential to guarantee patient safety. In addition, continuous training of the healthcare team, the use of technologies such as computerised systems and effective communication between professionals are essential to prevent errors (Santos et al., 2020; Freire et al., 2020).

Enteral drug administration presents specific challenges, such as the need to ensure the correct administration of drugs, proper hygiene of the fallopian tubes and the prevention of complications. The development of specific protocols for the administration of drugs by enteral feeding tube is crucial to ensure treatment efficacy and patient safety (Freire et al., 2020; Gama et al., 2019).

To summarise, the safe administration of medicines requires observance of the "nine rights", adequate preparation, staff training, use of technology and effective communication. By following these principles and adopting safety measures, healthcare professionals can ensure the administration of effective, safe and quality medicines to patients, contributing to the promotion of patient safety and excellence in healthcare.

The "right nine" include:

1. **Right Patient:** Verify the identity of the patient to ensure that the medicine is administered to the correct person.
2. **Correct medication:** Confirm that the prescribed medication is the one being administered.
3. **Correct dose:** Measure out the appropriate amount of medicine as prescribed.
4. **Correct route:** Ensure that the medicine is administered by the correct route (oral, intravenous, etc.).
5. **The right time:** Administer the medication at the right time, following the prescribed time.
6. Expiry Date: Check that the medicine is within its expiry date and in suitable condition for use.
7. **Correct recording: Correctly** document the administration of the medicine in the patient's file.
8. **Correct Action:** Understand and explain to the patient the expected action of the medication.

9. **Right Answer: Monitor** and evaluate the patient's response to the drug to ensure efficacy and safety.

1.3 Application of Virginia Henderson's Principles in Therapeutic Management

Virginia Henderson, one of the most influential nursing theorists, proposed a model of care that emphasises the importance of the nurse's independent role in patient care. Her principles focus on individualised and comprehensive care, covering not only the physical, but also the psychological, social and spiritual needs of the patient. The integration of Virginia Henderson's principles, which emphasise independence and respect for the dignity of the patient, is crucial in the management of the therapeutic regime, ensuring that treatment is not only limited to the physical aspects of the illness, but also considers the emotional, social and spiritual needs of patients, guaranteeing the safe and effective administration of therapy.
Henderson's principles suggest that nursing should ensure that patients are able to fulfil their basic needs in a way that preserves their dignity and integrity. This is directly reflected in the administration of medication in various ways:

- **Individualisation of care:** Each treatment plan must be adapted to the patient's individual characteristics, including their medical history, socioeconomic conditions and personal preferences. This ensures that medication is administered more effectively and with less risk of errors.
- **Patient Education and Empowerment:** Teaching patients about their medication regime is fundamental. The nurse should clearly explain the purpose and expected effects of the medication, as well as possible adverse effects, encouraging the patient to actively participate in their care plan.
- **Holistic support:** As well as focusing on the disease and its direct treatment, Henderson values supporting the emotional, social and spiritual needs of the patient, recognising that all these aspects are crucial to recovery and well-being.

Implementing the Principles in Clinical Practice

- **Effective communication:** Clear and empathetic communication is crucial to understanding the patient's concerns and expectations. This allows for a better assessment of needs and adaptation of nursing interventions, resulting in greater adherence to treatment.
- **Ongoing assessment:** Regular assessments are needed to adjust treatment as necessary, ensuring that care remains relevant and effective as the patient's condition evolves.
- **Promoting Autonomy:** Nurses should encourage and facilitate as much as possible the patient's independence in managing their own health, reinforcing education and self-care.

Challenges and Solutions

Implementing Henderson's principles can face a number of challenges, especially in acute care settings where the pace is fast and resources are often limited. Some solutions include:

- **Professional Training:** Frequent training and educational updates for nurses help keep care practices in line with the highest standards of safety and effectiveness.
- **Assistive technology:** Technological tools can assist in the monitoring and management of care, helping to personalise treatment and keep accurate and up-to-date records.
- **Organisational Culture:** Promoting a culture that values a patient-centred approach and evidence-based practice is the key to fully integrating Henderson's principles into the daily administration of medicines.

Chapter 2: Fundamentals of Nursing Pharmacology

The administration of medicines is one of the most critical responsibilities in nursing practice, requiring in-depth knowledge of pharmacology, precise preparation and administration techniques and the strict implementation of safety protocols to guarantee the patient's well-being.

2.1 The Importance of Understanding Pharmacokinetics and Pharmacodynamics in Nursing Practice

Pharmacology is the study of drug interactions with biological systems. For nurses, understanding pharmacokinetics (how the body affects the drug) and pharmacodynamics (how the drug affects the body) is essential.

This includes knowledge about how drugs are absorbed, distributed, metabolised and excreted, as well as their mechanisms of action, therapeutic effects and potential adverse effects. An understanding of pharmacokinetics and pharmacodynamics is crucial to the safe and effective practice of drug administration. The choice of models for pharmacokinetic studies and the interpretation of data must take into account genetic factors, gender, patient age, liver disease and drug interactions. In addition, pharmacokinetics and pharmacodynamics play a key role in understanding the drug use profile of different groups, such as the elderly, outpatients, rural residents and others. This understanding is crucial for the safe and effective practice of drug administration. The choice of models for pharmacokinetic studies and the interpretation of data must take into account genetic factors, gender, patient age, liver disease and drug interactions (Zamboni 2023; Ladebo et al., 2019).

Pharmacokinetics

Absorption

Absorption is the first step in the pharmacokinetic process, where the drug is transferred from the injection site to the bloodstream. The absorption rate and efficiency are influenced by a number of factors, including:

- **Route of administration:** Oral drugs can be affected by the presence of food, gastric pH and gastrointestinal motility. Injectable drugs (subcutaneous, intramuscular) bypass the gastrointestinal tract and can be absorbed more quickly.
- **Drug characteristics:** Solubility, chemical stability and formulation of the drug determine its ability to cross cell membranes.

Distribution

After absorption, the drug is distributed throughout the body, which is crucial for its effectiveness. Distribution depends on:

- **Protein binding:** Drugs can bind to plasma proteins, which influences their distribution in tissues.
- **Cellular barriers:** The ability of a drug to cross barriers such as the blood-brain barrier can determine its effectiveness in certain areas, such as the brain.

Metabolism

Metabolism transforms the drug into more water-soluble forms to facilitate excretion. This takes place mainly in the liver, through specific enzymes that chemically modify the drug. Understanding metabolism is vital to avoiding toxicity and drug interactions.

Excretion

The last phase of pharmacokinetics is the excretion of metabolites through various systems:

- **Renal:** The main route of excretion for many drugs and their metabolites, which occurs through glomerular filtration and tubular secretion.
- **Biliary and faecal:** Some drugs are excreted intact or as metabolites in the bile and eliminated in the faeces.

Pharmacodynamics

Mechanisms of action

Medicines can interact with the body in various ways:

- **Receptors:** Many drugs work by binding to specific receptors, modulating cellular activity. For example, beta-antagonists block adrenergic receptors in the heart, reducing blood pressure.
- **Enzymes:** Others inhibit or activate specific enzymes, affecting metabolic or biochemical processes in the body.

Therapeutic and adverse effects

Therapeutic effects are those that are desired, while adverse effects are unintended and often harmful. The relationship between the dose of the drug and the patient's response is fundamental to understanding both effects.

Response to drug dose

Drug Dose Response deals with the pharmacokinetic actions and mechanisms by which drugs act.

The intervals of action of the drug depend on the onset of action of the drug, the maximum action, and the duration of the effect.

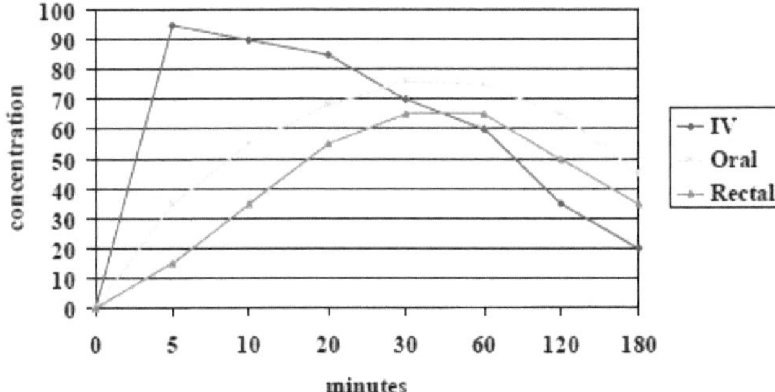

Dose-response curves:

- **Linear:** Gradual increases in dose result in proportional increases in response up to a certain point.
- **Saturation:** Increasing the dose beyond a certain point does not result in greater efficacy and can increase the risk of toxicity.

These curves help determine the ideal dose to achieve the desired effect with minimal adverse effects. Graphical visualisation of these curves provides an intuitive understanding of dose-response relationships and is essential for planning the therapeutic regimen.

2.2 Therapeutic classification of drugs

The therapeutic classification of drugs is a system used to organise drugs based on the conditions or diseases they treat. This system is fundamental for healthcare professionals, including nurses, pharmacists and doctors, as it facilitates the identification and selection of suitable drugs for specific treatments. Below, we'll discuss how drugs are categorised and some examples of common therapeutic classes.

1. Based on the disease or condition being treated: Medicines are often grouped according to the diseases or conditions for which they are most commonly prescribed. This approach helps healthcare professionals to quickly select an effective therapy based on the patient's condition.

2. Mechanism of action In addition to the target disease, medicines can also be classified by their mechanism of action, i.e. how they act in the body to exert their effects. This classification is particularly useful for understanding drug interactions and potential side effects.

Examples of Therapeutic Classes

1. Antihypertensives : These drugs are used to treat hypertension (high blood pressure). Within this class, there are several subcategories based on mechanisms of action, including ACE inhibitors, angiotensin II receptor blockers, diuretics, beta-blockers and calcium antagonists.

2. Antidiabetics : Medicines used to control and treat diabetes mellitus. Subcategories include insulins, insulin secretagogues (such as sulphonylureas and glinides), insulin sensitisers (such as biguanides and thiazolidinediones) and digestive enzyme inhibitors (such as alpha-glucosidase inhibitors).

3. Antibiotics Used to treat bacterial infections. Antibiotics can be categorised into classes such as penicillins, cephalosporins, macrolides, quinolones and tetracyclines, each of which is effective against different types of bacteria.

4. Antidepressants : Intended for the treatment of depressive disorders and associated conditions. These include selective serotonin reuptake inhibitors (SSRIs), tricyclic antidepressants, monoamine oxidase inhibitors (MAOIs) and atypical antidepressants.

5. Anti-inflammatories These include non-steroidal anti-inflammatory drugs (NSAIDs) and corticosteroids, which are used to reduce inflammation, pain and fever. They are commonly prescribed for conditions such as arthritis, injuries and autoimmune diseases.

Importance of Therapeutic Classification

Therapeutic classification not only simplifies the process of prescribing and dispensing medicines, but also helps with patient education and health management. Understanding therapeutic classes allows healthcare providers to anticipate potential side effects, better manage drug interactions and personalise treatments to meet patients' individual needs.

2.3 Therapeutic indications and types of therapeutic effects

The therapeutic indication for a medicine refers to the specific use or clinical condition for which the medicine is prescribed. Understanding the therapeutic indication is crucial to ensuring that the treatment is appropriate and effective. Therapeutic effects, on the other hand, are the desired benefits that a drug produces to treat or prevent a disease or symptom. Below, we'll break down these concepts and discuss the different types of therapeutic effects.

Therapeutic indication

Definition: The therapeutic indication of a medicine is the use for which it has been approved by the regulatory authorities, based on scientific evidence of its efficacy and safety. These indications are specified on the drug's label and in clinical treatment guidelines.

Examples:

- **Antibiotics:** Indicated for the treatment of specific bacterial infections.
- **Antihypertensives:** Used to reduce and control high blood pressure.
- **Antidepressants:** Prescribed for the treatment of depressive disorders and, in some cases, anxiety disorders.

Types of drug effects

Therapeutic effects

The therapeutic effect is the expected or predictable physiological response generated by a drug. The same drug can have several therapeutic effects.

The therapeutic effects of medicines can be classified into several categories, depending on their impact on the body and the disease being treated:

Bandages: These effects are intended to cure the disease or condition. For example, antibiotics that eradicate bacterial infections provide a curative effect by eliminating the underlying cause of the illness.

Palliative: Palliative effects do not treat the cause of the illness, but relieve the symptoms, improving the patient's quality of life. Medicines such as analgesics and antiemetics, which relieve pain and nausea respectively, are considered palliative.

Prophylactic or Preventive: These effects aim to prevent the occurrence of a disease or condition. Vaccines and preventive medicines for cardiovascular diseases, such as statins, are examples of agents with prophylactic effects.

Substitutes: These include medicines that replace substances or elements that are lacking in the body. For example, insulin is used in patients with type 1 diabetes to replace the insulin that the body cannot produce.

Disease Modifiers: Medicines that can alter the course of a chronic disease. Many treatments for autoimmune diseases, such as rheumatoid arthritis, are considered disease modifiers because they can slow down or modify the progression of the condition.

Knowledge of the types of therapeutic effects is essential for healthcare professionals when prescribing medicines, as it allows for better selection and management of treatment, ensuring that patients receive the most appropriate therapy for their condition. In addition, understanding these effects helps with patient education, allowing them to have realistic expectations about the results of treatment and to be aware of how medicines will help manage their health conditions.

Side effects

Side effects are unintended responses to a drug that occur when the drug is administered in normal doses. These effects are generally predictable and often described during the clinical trial phase of drug development.

Nurses must be able to identify and manage common side effects to minimise patient discomfort and optimise adherence to treatment. For example, when administering opiates, it is vital to monitor signs of excessive drowsiness and constipation, intervening if necessary with measures such as adjusting the dose or prescribing laxatives.

Adverse effects

Adverse effects are harmful and unexpected reactions to a drug that do not correspond to the intended pharmacological effect. They can vary in severity and, in some cases, be serious enough to require discontinuation of the drug.

The role of nursing is crucial in monitoring and responding promptly to adverse effects. Nurses should carry out detailed patient assessments before administering the drug, check for a history of allergies to the drug and watch carefully for signs of toxicity or allergic reactions. They should also educate patients about the warning signs of serious adverse effects so that they can seek medical help immediately.

Toxic effects

Toxic effects occur when exposure to a drug exceeds safe therapeutic levels, which can be due to overdose, accumulation due to organ dysfunction (such as kidney or liver failure), or harmful drug interactions.

Managing toxic effects involves close monitoring of vital functions and laboratory parameters to detect early signs of toxicity. Nurses must be proficient in emergency interventions, such as administering antidotes (when available) and basic life support. In addition, educating patients on the importance of following prescriptions and not exceeding recommended doses is fundamental.

2.4 Types of drug reactions: Idiosyncratic reactions and allergic reactions

In the context of pharmacology, it is essential for nurses to understand the types of drug reactions, especially idiosyncratic and allergic reactions, in order to effectively monitor patients and intervene appropriately. Here is a detailed breakdown of these reactions:

Idiosyncratic reactions

Definition: Idiosyncratic reactions are atypical responses to drugs that are not based on the known pharmacological action of the drug and cannot be predicted by the toxicological or pharmacodynamic profile of the drug. These reactions occur rarely and are unpredictable, often occurring regardless of the dose administered.

Mechanism: Although the exact mechanisms often remain unknown, idiosyncratic reactions are believed to involve genetic factors that alter drug metabolism, immune function or cellular response. These reactions can be triggered by enzyme deficiencies, genetic variations in metabolic pathways or immune abnormalities.

Examples:

- A patient may experience excessive sedation or agitation after taking an antihistamine, contrary to the usual expected effect.
- Serious idiosyncratic reactions can include agranulocytosis with antithyroid drugs or aplastic anaemia with some antibiotics.

Nurses should be aware of the potential for idiosyncratic reactions and educate patients on the importance of promptly reporting any atypical response. Careful monitoring, especially after the administration of new drugs, is crucial for the early detection of abnormalities.

Allergic reactions

Definition: Allergic drug reactions are adverse immune responses that occur when the body's immune system mistakenly identifies a drug component as a harmful antigen. These reactions can range from mild to severe and are more common with certain types of medication.

Mechanism: The reaction begins when the sensitised immune system responds to the drug by producing specific antibodies (typically IgE). On subsequent exposure to the same drug, these antibodies recognise and bind to the drug, triggering the release of chemical mediators such as histamine, which cause the symptoms of an allergic reaction.

Examples:

- Mild reactions include rash, hives and itching.
- Serious reactions can include anaphylaxis, characterised by difficulty breathing, swelling of the throat, tachycardia and potentially shock.

Nurses should carefully screen for a history of drug allergies before administering any medication. In the event of an allergic reaction, it is essential to immediately stop administering the suspected drug and start treatment for the allergic reaction, which may include the administration of adrenaline and respiratory support, depending on the severity.

Both idiosyncratic and allergic reactions require vigilance, knowledge and readiness on the part of nurses to ensure patient safety and the effectiveness of drug treatment. Continuing education in pharmacology and adverse drug reactions is vital to keep nurses up to date on the best practices for managing such reactions.

2.6 Drug interactions

A drug interaction occurs when the efficacy or toxicity of a drug is altered by the concomitant administration of another medicine, food, drink or environmental chemicals.

This phenomenon can result from interference with pharmacodynamics (the effect of the drug on the body) or pharmacokinetics (the way the drug is absorbed, distributed, metabolised or excreted by the body).

Drug interactions are not just limited to combinations between prescribed medicines; they can also involve over-the-counter medicines, food supplements, food and even drinks such as alcohol. For example, ingesting grapefruit juice can affect the metabolism of certain drugs in the liver, increasing the concentration of the drug in the blood and potentially its toxic effects.

Types of Drug Interaction Results

The outcome of a drug interaction can vary greatly depending on the substances involved:

1. **Intensifying the effect:**
    - It can include the intensification of desired effects or the manifestation of toxic effects.
    - For example, combining anticoagulant drugs with non-steroidal anti-inflammatory drugs can significantly increase the risk of bleeding.
2. **Decreased effects:**
    - One drug can reduce the effectiveness of another, leading to an insufficient therapeutic response.
    - A classic example is the reduced effectiveness of oral contraceptives when taken concomitantly with some antibiotics.
3. **New effects appear:**
    - In certain cases, the interaction can lead to the emergence of a new effect that is not observed when each drug is used alone.
    - This phenomenon can occur due to complex biochemical interactions between drugs and biological systems.

Three basic types of drug interactions

1. **Addition of Synergism:**
    - The combined effect of two drugs is exactly equal to the sum of the effects of each drug taken alone.
    - For example, the combination of two painkillers, such as paracetamol and ibuprofen, can provide better pain relief equivalent to the sum of their individual effects.

2. **Potentiation Synergism:**
    - The combined effect is greater than the sum of the effects of the drugs when used separately.
    - One example is the combination of an angiotensin-converting enzyme (ACE) inhibitor and a diuretic, which work together to reduce blood pressure more effectively than when each is used alone.
3. **Antagonism:**
    - One drug reduces or cancels out the effect of another.
    - This can be seen, for example, in the concomitant administration of a beta-agonist such as salbuterol, which dilates the bronchi, and a beta-blocker, which can reduce or cancel out this effect.

Drug interactions represent a complex aspect of drug management, requiring healthcare professionals, especially nurses, to be constantly vigilant and to have in-depth knowledge of the pharmacological properties of drugs. Continuous education on drug interactions is essential to ensure patient safety and treatment efficacy, facilitating the early identification of potential interactions and the implementation of strategies to mitigate their adverse effects.

2.7 Tolerance to drug use or habituation

Drug tolerance, also known as habituation, is a pharmacological phenomenon in which the response to a drug decreases after repeated use, leading to the need for progressively higher doses to achieve the effect originally obtained with lower doses. This phenomenon is particularly relevant in the management of long-term treatments and can affect the efficacy and safety of the therapeutic regime.

Definition and Tolerance Mechanisms

1Pharmacodynamic tolerance: refers to the decreased response to the effects of a drug due to adaptive changes in cell signalling systems or target receptors. For example, with continued use of opioids, neuronal receptors can become less sensitive to the drug, requiring higher doses to achieve pain relief.

Pharmacokinetic (metabolic) tolerance: Occurs when repeated use of a drug increases the body's ability to metabolise it, often due to enzyme induction in the liver. This results in a reduction in the concentration of the active drug available in the body, decreasing its effectiveness.

Tissue tolerance: Some tissues can become less reactive to a drug after prolonged exposure, without changes in signalling mechanisms or metabolism. This can be seen in cases such as nitroglycerin therapy for angina, where the vasodilator effect decreases with continued use.

Clinical implications of drug tolerance

Dose adjustment and monitoring: The development of tolerance may require periodic dose adjustments to maintain therapeutic efficacy without compromising patient safety. Nurses and doctors should carefully monitor for signs of tolerance and adjust treatment as necessary.

Risk of dependence and abuse: In some cases, especially with opioid analgesics or sedatives, tolerance can lead to an increased risk of dependence and abuse, as patients may seek higher or more frequent doses of the drug to achieve the same effect.

Weaning and Medication Rotation Planning: To avoid the negative effects of tolerance, especially with pain medications or anxiolytics, it may be necessary to implement drug weaning or rotation strategies. This involves periodically replacing one drug with another with a different mechanism of action to reduce tolerance and minimise the risks of adverse effects.

Chapter 3: Administering the Medication Regimen: Meaning, Settings and Basic Principles

The administration of the medication regime involves the proper management of the patient's medication, ensuring that the patient receives the right medicines, in the right doses, by the right methods and at the right times. This process is crucial for maximising therapeutic efficacy and minimising the risks of adverse effects, drug interactions and other complications.

Administration Environments

The administration of the medication regime can take place in various scenarios, each with specific characteristics and requirements:

1. **Home care:** In this context, the administration of medication is often carried out by the patient themselves or by family carers, under the guidance of healthcare professionals. The focus is on ensuring adherence to the therapeutic regime in an environment outside a healthcare unit.
2. **Differentiated Care: This** includes hospitals and specialised clinics where the administration of medicines is carried out by trained healthcare professionals. This environment allows for stricter control and constant monitoring of the therapeutic regime.
3. **Primary Health Care:** Involves the functional units of primary health care where medicines are administered for long-term treatment or chronic conditions, with an emphasis on disease prevention and management.

3.1 Basic principles

The effective administration of the drug regime is based on several basic principles that guarantee the safety and efficacy of the treatment:

1. **Knowledge of Medicines:**
    - Understand the drug's actions, effects, contraindications and side effects.
    - Knowledge of specific characteristics, such as generic name, trade name, usual dose, route of administration and expiry date.
2. **Preparation of medicines:**

- Checking the preparation environment to minimise distractions and errors.
- Respect for the specific preparation and administration techniques for each type of medicine.

3. **Medication Administration:**
    - Compliance with the "right nine": right patient, right medicine, right dose, right route, right time, right action, right form of presentation, right answer and right documentation.
    - Monitoring and surveillance of the patient to assess the response to the drug.
4. **Education and Communication:**
    - Inform the patient about the name of the medicine, the purpose, the intended effect and possible side effects.
    - Check for allergies and respect the patient's right to refuse medication.
5. **Rigorous documentation:**
    - Effective recording of all medicines administered, including details such as dose, route of administration, time and relevant observations.
    - Documentation of any refusal of medication and the reasons for it.

Medication administration is a critical responsibility in nursing practice, requiring a comprehensive understanding of medications and effective communication with patients to ensure that treatments are carried out safely and effectively.

3.2 Prescribing and calculating drug doses

Prescribing and converting medicines are essential processes in medical and nursing practice, involving the determination of suitable medicines and their doses, as well as adjustments to these doses or changes of medicines when necessary. These processes require in-depth knowledge of pharmacology, the patient's individual needs and drug interactions in order to guarantee the effectiveness and safety of treatment.

Prescription medicines

Prescribing medicines is the process by which doctors and other qualified healthcare professionals (such as some specialist nurses, depending on the legislation) select and authorise the use of specific medicines to treat a patient's medical conditions.

Fundamental principles:

- **Clinical Assessment:** Includes examination of the patient's health conditions, medical history and any current treatment to identify the most appropriate medication.
- **Determining the dose: Based on the** patient's weight, age, kidney and liver function, among other clinical factors.
- **Consideration of Interactions:** Evaluation of potential drug interactions is essential to avoid adverse effects.
- **Patient information:** It is essential to provide clear information on the use, benefits and potential risks of prescription medicines.

Calculating the drug dose

Calculating drug doses is a critical aspect of nursing practice, essential for ensuring the safety and efficacy of pharmacological treatment. Errors in dose calculation can lead to adverse clinical outcomes, including underdosing or overdosing, with potentially serious consequences for patients.

Factors to consider:

- **Body weight:** Many drug doses are calculated based on the patient's body weight, especially for drugs with narrow therapeutic margins, such as antibiotics and chemotherapy.
- **Age:** Age can affect the pharmacokinetics and pharmacodynamics of drugs. For example, infants and the elderly may require dosage adjustments due to differences in drug metabolism and excretion.
- **Renal and hepatic function:** Renal and hepatic function can significantly affect how a drug is metabolised and excreted. Patients with renal or hepatic impairment may require lower doses or adjustments to the interval between doses.
- **Medical conditions:** Conditions such as obesity, pregnancy and concomitant diseases can influence dosage requirements and the choice of medication.

Calculation Methods:

- **Dose per unit weight:** The dose is often calculated on the basis of milligrams of the drug per kilogram of the patient's body weight.
- **Body Surface Area Based Dose:** Used for some oncological drugs, where the dose is calculated based on the patient's body surface area, derived from formulas that include weight and height.

Basic steps for calculating drug doses

1. **Determine the prescribed dose:**
    - Start by identifying the total dose prescribed by your doctor, which is usually expressed in milligrams (mg), micrograms (mcg) or international units (IU).
2. **Check the concentration of the medicine available:**
    - Check the concentration of the drug available in the unit. This concentration can be expressed in mg/ml, mcg/ml, or IU/ml, depending on the drug.
3. **Calculate the volume required for administration:**
    - Use the formula:

      $$\text{required volume} = \frac{\text{Prescribed dose}}{\text{Drug concentration}}$$

    - For example, if the prescribed dose is 100 mg and the concentration of the drug available is 50 mg/ml, the volume needed will be:

$$\text{required volume} = \frac{100\ \text{mg}}{50\ \text{mg/ml}} = 2\text{ml}$$

4. **Adjustments based on patient factors:**
    - Consider any patient-specific factors that may influence the dose, such as body weight, age, kidney and liver function.
    - For medicines that require weight-based adjustment, the dose can be calculated as:

Dosage by weight = Specific dose *Patient weight

- Adjust the dose as necessary based on clinical assessment and pharmacological recommendations.

Principles of Safe Calculation

- **Clarity of the prescription:** Make sure that all prescriptions are clear and complete. If in doubt, it is crucial to check with the doctor before administering the medicine.
- **Use of tools and resources: Use** standard dose calculators and reference tables to check calculated doses, especially for high-risk drugs.
- **Double Check:** Practise double checking with another healthcare professional for all calculated doses, especially for medicines that have narrow therapeutic margins or are administered in critical situations.
- **Proper documentation:** Meticulously record the calculated dose, the calculation method used and any other relevant information to ensure continuity and safety of care.

Chapter 4: Therapeutic routes of administration

Therapeutic routes of administration refer to the different methods by which medicines are administered to the body to treat, prevent or diagnose diseases. The choice of route of administration is crucial to the effectiveness of treatment and is determined by factors such as the nature of the drug, the condition of the patient, how quickly the drug needs to work and the desired duration of the effect. Below, we explore the main routes of administration and their characteristics.

1. Oral

Description: Oral administration is the most common, involving the ingestion of medication by mouth.

Advantages:

- Convenient and comfortable for the patient.
- Ideal for long-term medication.

Disadvantages:

- Absorption can be affected by the presence of food, stomach pH and other medicines.
- Not suitable for unconscious or vomiting patients.

2. Parenteral

Description: Includes all routes that bypass the gastrointestinal tract, such as intravenous, intramuscular and subcutaneous.

- **Intravenous (IV) route:** Direct administration into a vein.
  - **Advantages:** Fast action and precise dosage control.
  - **Disadvantages:** Requires strict aseptic technique, risk of infection and rapid adverse reactions.
- **Intramuscular (IM):** Injection into the muscle.
  - **Advantages:** Faster absorption than the subcutaneous route.
  - **Disadvantages:** Can be painful, risk of damage to nerves or blood vessels.
- **Subcutaneous (SC):** Injection into the tissue beneath the skin.
  - **Advantages:** Easier and less painful than IM, suitable for slow and continuous administration.

- **Disadvantages:** Limited volume that can be administered, risk of irritation at the injection site.

3. Topic

Description: Application of drugs to the skin or mucous membranes.

Advantages:

- Local effects with less risk of systemic effects.
- Use in dermatological, ophthalmological and other treatments.

Disadvantages:

- Variable absorption and sometimes ineffective for systemic effects.
- Risk of local allergic reactions.

4. Respiratory (inhaled)

Description: Administration of drugs by inhalation into the lungs.

Advantages:

- Fast-acting, especially for lung diseases such as asthma or COPD.
- Lower dosage required compared to oral, reducing side effects.

Disadvantages:

- Need for specific devices and proper inhalation technique.
- Risk of airway irritation.

5. Other routes

- **Rectal:** Suppositories or enemas.
- **Sublingual:** Absorption through the tissues under the tongue or mouth.
- **Ophthalmology:** Eye drops or ointments for eye diseases.
- **Otological:** Ear drops for the treatment of ear infections or conditions.
- **Nasal: Nasal** sprays or drops for sinus or systemic conditions.

The choice of route of administration is a crucial clinical decision that must take into account efficacy, safety, convenience and patient comfort. Healthcare professionals, especially nurses, must be familiar with the advantages and disadvantages of each route in order to optimise the therapeutic regime and guarantee the best results for patients.

4.1 Procedure for administering oral medication

Administering oral medication is one of the most common tasks carried out by nurses. Following a standard procedure not only guarantees patient safety, but also maximises the effectiveness of treatment. Below, I present a step-by-step guide based on the guidelines of the nursing procedures manual of the Central Administration of the Health System (ACSS) and other evidence available in the document provided.

Step-by-Step Administration of Oral Medication

1. **Preparing for Administration:**
    - **Check the prescription:** Confirm the patient's name, the medication prescribed, the dosage, the route of administration and the time of administration.
    - **Hand hygiene:** Wash your hands before handling any medication to prevent the transmission of infections.
    - **Prepare the medication:** Use aseptic techniques to prepare the required dose. Check the medication three times against the prescription to ensure accuracy.
2. **Nine Rights Check:**
    - **Right patient:** confirm the patient's identity using at least two unique identifiers (such as name and date of birth) before administering medication.
    - Check each element with the prescription to avoid medication errors.
3. **Medication Administration:**
    - **Inform and educate the patient:** Explain the name of the medicine, what it is for, how it should be taken and possible side effects.
    - **Administer the medication:** Give the patient the medication with a glass of water, observing them while they take the medication to ensure that it is taken correctly.
4. **Post-administration monitoring:**
    - **Watch out for adverse reactions:** Monitor the patient for any effects after administration, especially if it is the first dose of the medicine.

- **Documentation:** Record the administration of the medicine in the patient's file, including the time and relevant observations on the patient's response.

5. **Continuous assessment:**
   - **Re-evaluate efficacy and safety:** Continue to monitor the efficacy of the treatment and any signs of adverse reactions in subsequent administrations.

This procedure is grounded in evidence-based practice that emphasises patient safety and the effectiveness of therapy. Checking the "right nine" is a critical safety standard to prevent medication errors, which are one of the most common sources of adverse events in healthcare. Patient education promotes adherence and allows patients to actively participate in their treatment, increasing the likelihood of positive therapeutic outcomes. Following a standardised procedure for administering oral medication ensures that the care provided is safe, effective and consistent with best nursing practice. A commitment to precision in the preparation and administration of medication, coupled with effective communication and careful monitoring, is essential to modern nursing practice.

4.2 Procedure for administering rectal medication

Rectal drug administration is a commonly used method to ensure effective drug absorption in patients who cannot take medication orally or in situations where the drug is more effective by this route.

Step-by-step for administering rectal medication

1. **Preparing for Administration:**
   - **Check the prescription: confirm** all the "right nine"
   - **Hand hygiene:** Hands should be sanitised before preparing the medication to minimise the risk of contamination.
   - **Prepare the medicine:** Make sure the medicine is in the correct form for rectal administration (such as suppositories, enemas or foams).
2. **Explanation and positioning of the patient:**

- **Inform the patient:** Explain the procedure, the reason for using this route and what to expect during administration.
- **Position the patient:** The patient should be positioned on their side with their legs slightly bent (Sims position), which facilitates administration and convenience.

3. **Medication Administration:**
   - **Use of gloves:** Wear gloves when administering the medicine.
   - **Lubrication:** Lubricate the tip of the suppository or the tip of the enema applicator to facilitate insertion.
   - **Insertion:** With one hand, spread the upper part of the buttock to expose the anus. With the other hand, hold the suppository by the rounded end and insert the tapered tip into the anus first.
   - **Adequate depth:** Insert the suppository gently, pushing it with your index finger until it is about 2.5 to 4 centimetres inside the rectum, which is usually enough to ensure that it is not expelled involuntarily.
4. **After administration:**
   - **Advise the patient:** Ask the patient to lie on their side for a few minutes after insertion to help keep the suppository in place and facilitate absorption of the medicine.
   - **Disposal and hygiene:** Remove gloves and dispose of them according to the hoapitalar waste sorting principle. Wash your hands again after the procedure.
5. **Documentation:**
   - **Record the procedure:** Document the administration of the suppository in the patient's file, including the time of administration and any relevant observations about the patient's response or difficulties encountered during the procedure.
6. **Continuous evaluation and monitoring:**
   - **Efficacy assessment:** Monitor the efficacy of the drug as absorbed from the rectal route, adjusting as necessary based on the patient's response and clinical conditions.

The rectal administration of medicines offers an important alternative when the oral route is not feasible. This route is particularly useful for medicines that require rapid absorption or are irritating to the stomach. The position of the Sims used during administration helps to maximise patient comfort and the effectiveness of drug absorption. Detailed documentation and monitoring are essential to ensure patient safety and treatment effectiveness, in line with evidence-based practices in nursing.

By using the standard procedure for administering medication rectally, nurses can ensure that the administration is carried out safely and effectively, while maintaining the dignity and comfort of the patient. This procedure helps to ensure that all critical aspects of drug administration are considered to maximise drug therapy and minimise risks.

4.3 Administration of otological medicines

The ear route refers to the administration of medication into the ear, generally used to treat conditions affecting the ear canal and middle ear. It is essential to follow a proper procedure to ensure that the treatment is effective and safe. Here are the detailed steps for administering medication via the ear route:

Preparing for Administration

1. **Check the prescription:**
    - Confirm the "right nine" before proceeding
2. **Hand hygiene:**
    - Wash your hands with soap and water before handling any medication to minimise the risk of infection.
3. **Use of gloves:**
    - Wear disposable gloves to maintain hygiene and protect both the professional and the patient.
4. **Prepare the medicine:**
    - make sure the medicine is at room temperature to avoid the discomfort that can be caused by a solution that is too cold or too hot.
5. **Positioning the patient:**
    - Ask the patient to tilt their head to the opposite side of the ear to be treated so that the affected ear is facing upwards. This facilitates the administration of the drug and allows it to properly reach the ear canal.

Medication Administration

6. **Cleaning the outer ear:**
    - If visible, clean any wax or discharge from the outer ear using gauze or a clean cloth. Avoid inserting any object into the ear canal.
7. **Application of the drug:**
    - Pull the ear to prepare the ear canal:
    - In **adults and children over 3 years old**, gently pull the ear up and back to align the ear canal.
    - In **children under 3 years of age**, pull the ear downwards and backwards.
    - **Apply the drops:** Hold the bottle in your dominant hand and apply the prescribed number of drops into the ear canal, without letting the tip of the applicator touch the ear or other surfaces to avoid contamination.
    - **Hold the position for a few minutes** to allow the drops to penetrate deep into the ear canal. You can gently massage the base of the ear to help distribute the medicine.

8. **After administration:**
    - Ask the patient to keep their head tilted for a few minutes to allow the drug to disperse properly through the ear canal.
    - If necessary, gently press the tragus (the small protrusion in front of the ear canal) several times to help get the medicine deeper into the ear.

Monitoring and Documentation

9. **Warning of side effects:**
    - Monitor the patient for any signs of irritation or allergic reaction and report any of these effects immediately.
10. **Documentation:**
    - Document the administration of the medicine, including the date, time, medicine administered and any relevant observations on the patient's condition and response to treatment.
11. **Patient education:**

- Instruct the patient on how to continue treatment at home, if applicable, and inform the patient of the necessary precautions to avoid contamination or worsening of the disease.

The otological administration of medication must be carried out with care and precision to ensure that the treatment is effective and comfortable for the patient. Following the appropriate steps helps prevent infection and ensures that the drug is optimally delivered to the desired site of action.

4.4 Administration of ophthalmic medicines

The administration of eye medication is a common procedure for treating various eye conditions, such as infections, inflammation, glaucoma and allergies. It is essential that the procedure is carried out correctly to ensure the effectiveness of the treatment and avoid contamination or injury to the eye. Here are the detailed steps for the safe administration of ophthalmic medicines, such as eye drops and ophthalmic ointments.

Step-by-Step Administration of Ophthalmological Medicines

1. Preparation

- **Wash your hands thoroughly** with soap and water to avoid transmitting germs to your eyes.
- **Check the medicine** to make sure it is the right one and note the expiry date.
- **Explain the procedure to** the patient, including what to expect during administration and how the medicine will help treat their eye disease.

2. Positioning the patient

- Ask the patient to tilt their head back or lie down, if possible. Ask them to look up.

3. Administration of eye drops

- **Cleaning: Wipe away** any discharge around the patient's eyes with a sterile gauze pad or clean cloth.
- **Prevention of contamination:** Hold the eye drops bottle without touching the tip to any surface, including the patient's skin or eyes.

- **Drop application:** With your other hand, gently pull the lower eyelid to create a small pocket. Sink the drops into the conjunctival sac, without allowing the applicator to touch the eye or eyelids.
- Ask the patient to blink gently to distribute the drops evenly.

4. Administration of ophthalmic ointments

- **Ointment application: As with eye** drops, pull the lower eyelid downwards. Apply a small strip of ointment to the conjunctival sac, from one corner of the eye to the other, avoiding touching the applicator to the eye.
- **Patient instructions:** The patient should close their eyes gently for 1 or 2 minutes and move their eyes in various directions to spread the ointment.

5. After administration

- **Cleaning:** Close the bottle or tube of ointment immediately after use to avoid contamination.
- **Final instructions:** Inform the patient to avoid rubbing their eyes after application and discuss any specific precautions related to the medicine.
- **Dispose of Materials: Dispose of** any gauze or materials used during the procedure.

6. Monitoring and documentation

- **Note:** The patient should be monitored for a few minutes after administration for any immediate adverse reactions.
- **Documentation:** Record the administration of the medicine in the patient's file, including the date, time and any relevant observations about the patient's condition and response to the medicine.

Important Tips

- Always wear gloves if the patient has infections.
- Never use the same bottle or tube for more than one patient to avoid cross-contamination.

The administration of ophthalmic medication requires precision and care to ensure patient safety and treatment efficacy. Following the appropriate steps and maintaining good hygiene practices are essential to avoid complications and promote the patient's ocular health.

4.5 Step-by-Step Administration of Inhaled Medicines

1. Preparation

- **Wash your hands** with soap and water to avoid contaminating the inhaler or the medicine.
- **Check the medicine** to make sure it's the right one, the right dosage, and note the expiry date.
- **Instruct the patient** about the procedure, explaining how the drug helps treat their respiratory condition.

2. Preparing the device

- **Make sure the inhaler is clean** and correctly assembled. If it is a metered dose inhaler (MDI), shake it well before use.
- **Check the inhaler charge**, if applicable, to make sure there is enough medicine for the dose.

3. Positioning the patient

- Ask the patient to sit or stand in a comfortable position that allows for deep, relaxed breathing.

4. Drug administration

- **Instructions for use of the metered dose inhaler (MDI):**
    - Ask the patient to exhale completely, moving the inhaler away from their mouth.
    - Place the inhaler in the patient's mouth, between the lips, closing tightly around the mouthpiece.
    - Ask the patient to start inhaling slowly and deeply and, at the same time, press the inhaler to release a dose of the medicine.
    - Hold your breath for 10 seconds, if possible, to allow the medicine to settle in your lungs.
    - Exhale slowly and relaxed.
- **Instructions for using nebulisers:**
    - Connect the nebuliser to the power supply and add the prescribed medicine to the nebuliser container.
    - Ask the patient to breathe normally through the mask or mouthpiece, allowing the medicated mist to be inhaled continuously until the end of the session, which usually lasts 5 to 10 minutes.

5. Post-administration

- **Inspect the inhaler** to ensure that all the medicine has been used or that the device is ready for the next use.
- **Instruct the patient** to rinse their mouth with water after using inhaled corticosteroids to prevent fungal infections in the mouth.
- **Cleaning the device: Clean** the inhaler mouthpiece with a dry cloth and store it according to the manufacturer's instructions.

6. Monitoring and documentation

- **Observe the patient** for any adverse reactions during and after administration.
- **Document the administration**, including the date, time and any relevant observations about the patient's condition and response to treatment.

Important Tips

- For patients using inhalers for the first time or who have difficulty with the technique, a spacer chamber can be recommended to improve the administration of the medicine.
- Ensure that the patient knows the proper inhalation technique and understands the importance of adhering to the treatment regime.

Administering medication by inhalation requires careful attention to technique to ensure that the drug reaches the lungs effectively. It is essential to follow the correct steps, educate the patient on the proper use of inhalers and monitor the effectiveness of the treatment to ensure the best possible management of respiratory conditions.

4.6 Preparation of injectable medication

The preparation of injectable medication involves the use of vials, usually made of glass, which are sealed with a rubber stopper and protected by a metal or plastic cap. This cap has a part that can be pierced by a needle to access the contents of the vial. Some vials are for single use, while others allow multiple doses and can be stored for a specific time under suitable conditions, such as refrigeration, after reconstitution.

Vials containing the active ingredient in powder form must be reconstituted with an appropriate solvent, which is usually sterile water or physiological saline. After reconstitution, these preparations should be used immediately or stored as recommended by the manufacturer to prevent degradation.
Ampoules are small sealed glass containers that are opened by breaking the neck of the ampoule and are intended for immediate use after opening to avoid contamination.

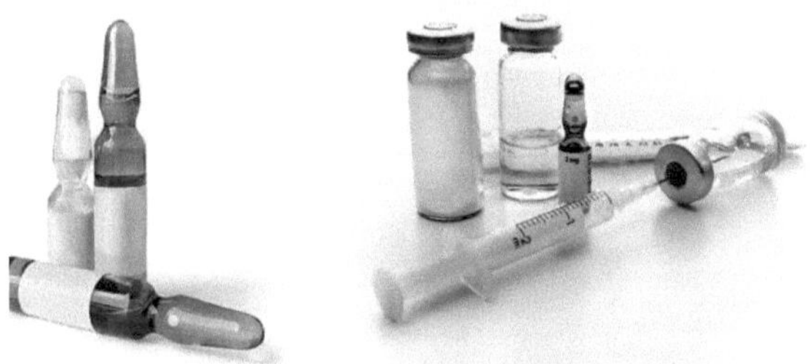

Ampoules and vials for injectable medicines

Parenteral medicines are prepared using a syringe and needle. The choice of syringe depends on the volume to be administered, with smaller syringes, such as insulin syringes, being used for volumes of less than 1 ml. These syringes have graduations that allow for precise dosing.

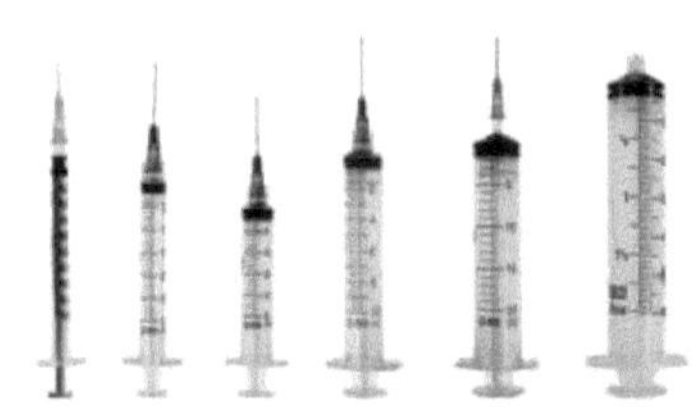

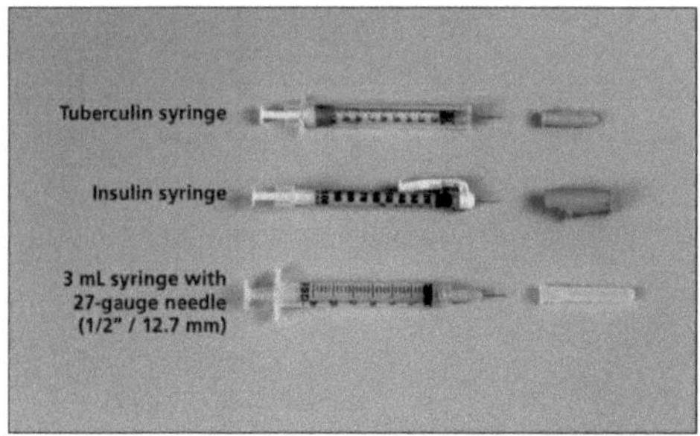

Needles for preparing and administering therapy are identified by the diameter of the lumen (gauge (G)) and the length of the needle (inches). The larger the "G", the smaller the lumen diameter, i.e. the thinner the needle.

Needles are selected based on their calibre and length. The choice of needle gauge depends on the viscosity of the medicine, while the length is adequate to ensure that the medicine is administered to the correct place in the body, avoiding excessive punctures that could hit unwanted muscles or nerves.

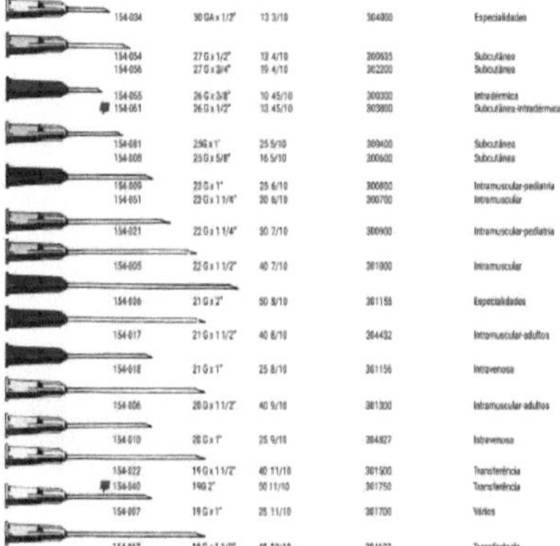

TABLE 1 - Examples of needles depending on size, length and route of administration

Length / Calibre	12 millimetres	16 millimetres	25 millimetres	30 millimetres	40 millimetres	50 millimetres
27G						
26G						
25G						
24G						
23G						
22G						
21G						
20G						
19G						

When preparing injections, it is essential to check the "clarity" of the drug, making sure there are no particles or changes in colour that could indicate contamination or instability of the product. After preparation, the injection should be administered following aseptic techniques to minimise the risk of infection.

4.7 Preparation and Administration of Intradermal Drugs (ID)

Intradermal (ID) drug administration is a procedure used mainly for allergy tests or to administer vaccines such as BCG. This method involves injecting a small amount of medicine directly into the dermis, which is the layer just below the surface of the skin.

Preparation for intradermal injection

1. **Selection and preparation of the injection site:**
    - The most common site for intradermal injection is the lower part of the forearm. The area should be selected because it is flat and free of lesions, visible veins, hair and bone.
    - Clean the area with an antiseptic, such as 70 per cent rubbing alcohol, to reduce the risk of infection. Allow the skin to dry completely before proceeding.
2. **Preparation of medicines:**
    - that the medicine is at room temperature for the patient's comfort.
    - Check the medicine for the correct dose, expiry date and clarity. Do not use if the solution is cloudy or contains precipitates.
    - Use a small syringe, usually 1 ml, with a fine needle, usually 25 to 27 gauge. Tuberculin syringes are often used because of their precision for small volumes.
3. **Aspiration technique:**
    - Aspirate the medicine as prescribed, ensuring that there are no air bubbles in the syringe, which could affect the accuracy of the dose administered.

Medication Administration

4. **Injection technique:**

- With the patient relaxed and the arm at rest, stretch the skin between the thumb and forefinger. This isolates the dermis and facilitates precise injection.
- Insert the needle into the skin at an angle of 10 to 15 degrees with the bevel facing upwards, inserting only the tip of the needle. A correct insertion should show minimal resistance.
- Inject the medicine slowly. A small blister (papule) should form on the skin, indicating that the drug is being administered in the correct place.

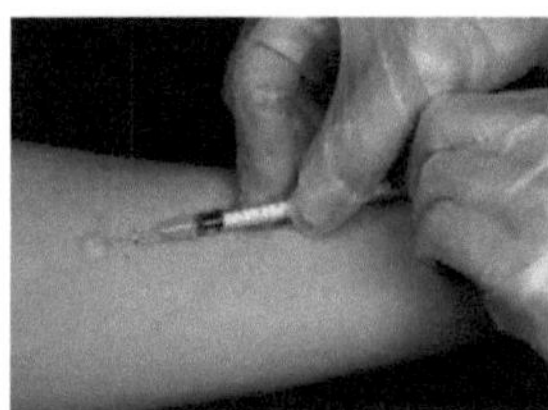

- Remove the needle and apply a dry gauze pad to the injection site to absorb any medication that may drip out when the needle is removed, but do not rub the area.

5. **Post-injection care:**
    - Observe the patient for a few minutes after the injection to detect any immediate adverse reactions.
    - Instruct the patient not to rub the injection site, which can disperse the drug and reduce its effectiveness.

Documentation and Monitoring

6. **Documentation:**
    - Record the administration, including the date, time, injection site, drug and dose administered, as well as the patient's response to the procedure.
7. **Monitoring:**
    - Monitor and document any local or systemic reactions in the days following administration, especially in allergy or tuberculin tests.

Intradermal drug administration requires precision and care to ensure that the drug is delivered correctly into the dermis. Following the correct preparation and administration steps, along with proper monitoring, is crucial for treatment efficacy and patient safety.

4.8 Preparation and administration of subcutaneous (SC) medicines

Subcutaneous (SC) drug administration is an effective method for administering drugs directly into the subcutaneous tissue, which is the layer of tissue just under the skin. This method is commonly used for the administration of vaccines, insulin and anticoagulants, among others. Here is a detailed guide to the safe preparation and administration of drugs by this route.

Subcutaneous injections are administered into the fatty tissue just below the skin layer. This method is often used to administer drugs such as insulin, anticoagulants and vaccines. Here is an illustrative guide to the most common sites for subcutaneous injections and the proper technique for administering them.

Frequent sites for subcutaneous injections

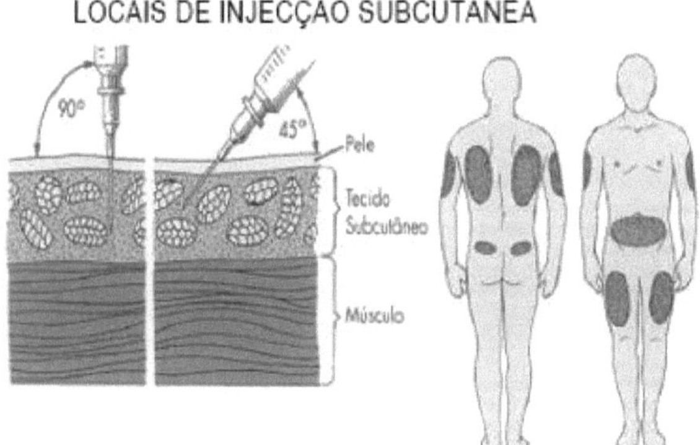

1. **Abdomen:**
    - The abdomen is the favoured site for subcutaneous injections due to its easy accessibility and large area of adipose tissue.
    - Avoid the area around the navel with a radius of approximately 5 cm.
2. **Upper arm:**
    - Use the area on the back of the arm, between the shoulder and the elbow. This area is generally less utilised, but is suitable due to the fatty tissue present.
3. **Thigh:**

- The front and outer thigh provide a good site for injections, especially for patients who administer their own injections, as it is easy to see and reach.

4. **Upper scapular region of the back:**
   - This area, just above and behind the waist, is less common, but can be used for people with less adipose tissue elsewhere.
5. **Flank:**
   - The flank area, just above the hips, is also a potential site, especially for obese patients, where other areas may be less accessible.

Preparation for subcutaneous injection

1. **Checking medication:**
   - Check the prescription for the "right nine" - the certainty of the patient, drug, dose, route, time, action, form, response and registration are correct.
   - make sure that the medicine is at the right temperature, especially if it is stored in the fridge.
2. **Choice of material:**
   - Use a small syringe, with 25 to 27 gauge needles, and an appropriate length to reach the subcutaneous tissue without hitting the muscle, usually between 12 and 16 mm.
3. **Preparation of the injection site:**
   - Select an appropriate injection site, such as the abdomen, upper arm, anterior thigh or upper scapular region of the back.
   - Clean the area with an antiseptic solution and leave to dry naturally to reduce the risk of infection.

Medication Administration

4. **Administration Technician:**
   - Hold the clean, dry skin, forming a skin fold, with one hand and with the other insert the needle quickly at an angle of 45 to 90 degrees, depending on the amount of adipose tissue that surrounds you and the length of the needle.

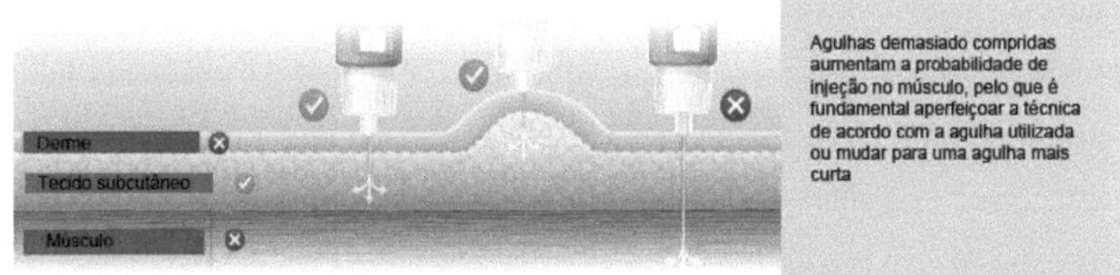

- Inject the medicine slowly and continuously. Do not reinsert the needle once it has been removed.

5. **After the injection:**
    - Do not massage the injection site to avoid irritation and dispersal of the drug.
    - If necessary, apply a light compress if there is minor bleeding.
6. **Safe Disposal:**
    - Dispose of needles and syringes in a sharps container in accordance with local safety guidelines.

Documentation and Monitoring

7. **Documentation:**
    - Document all the details of the administration, including the date, time, exact place of injection, the drug, the dose and any reaction from the patient.
8. **Patient monitoring:**
    - Monitor the patient for any local or systemic adverse reactions, especially the first few times the drug is administered.
    - Evaluate the effectiveness of the medicine as indicated, monitoring the patient's symptoms or carrying out follow-up tests as necessary.

Special considerations

- In patients receiving frequent injections, such as those being treated with insulin, it is important to alternate injection sites to avoid lipodystrophy, which is the loss of local fat tissue that can affect the absorption of the drug.
- Make sure you educate the patient and/or carers on how to administer injections safely and effectively, especially if the treatment is prolonged.

Subcutaneous drug administration is a common procedure that requires proper technique and specific knowledge to guarantee the safety and efficacy of the treatment. Following these guidelines not only helps prevent complications, but also ensures that the patient receives the maximum therapeutic benefit from the drug administered.

4.9. Preparation and Administration of Drugs by Intramuscular (IM) Route

Drugs are administered intramuscularly (IM) when you are looking for rapid absorption of the drug (15 to 20 minutes) and a long-lasting effect. The amount of medication that can be administered varies according to the capacity of the muscle to accommodate the volume, which can vary from 1ml to 5ml in adults, depending on the muscle chosen. In children, the acceptable volumes are lower.

The drug is injected into a dense area of the muscle, which allows larger volumes to be accommodated due to the accelerated absorption of the drug into the bloodstream, benefiting from the high number of muscle fibres present in this area.

IM injections tend to be less painful when applied correctly and are suitable for administering concentrated, irritating drugs that can damage the subcutaneous tissue. It is essential to be vigilant and aware of the possible complications related to the administration of drugs by this route, especially due to the rapid systemic absorption that can intensify these risks, including anaphylactic reactions. As a precaution, it is recommended that patients undergoing outpatient administration of IM medication remain in the healthcare facility for a minimum of 30 minutes after the injection.

Improper choice of injection site and technical errors can increase the risk of pain, nerve damage, haemorrhage, accidental intravenous administration and the formation of sterile abscesses, particularly if injections are repeatedly carried out at the same site with poor blood circulation.

Sites of intramuscular administration

The site chosen for an intramuscular injection depends on a number of factors, including the type of drug, the volume of the dose, the patient's age and physical condition. There is some discrepancy in the guidelines on recommended injection sites, making clinical judgement essential for each specific case.

Muscle Groups for Intramuscular Injection

The most common sites for intramuscular injections are divided into three main muscle groups:

1. **Deltoid muscle:**

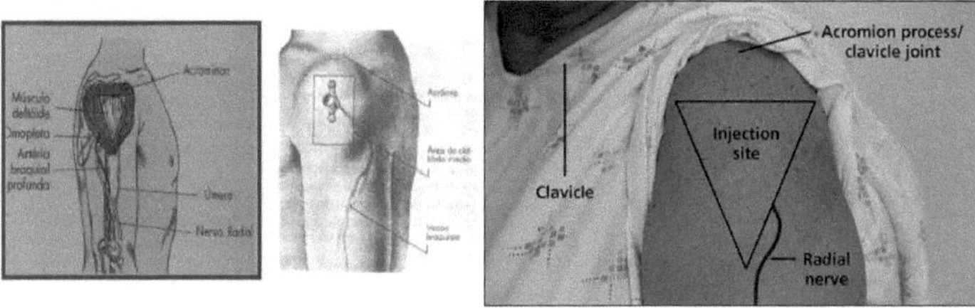

- Location: Upper arm.
- Use: Preferably used for the administration of small volumes, such as vaccines, due to its easy accessibility in various body positions.
- Limitations: Due to the relatively small muscle area, there are restrictions on the number of injections and the volume that can be administered on each occasion.

2. **Gluteal muscles (dorsogluteal and ventrogluteal):**

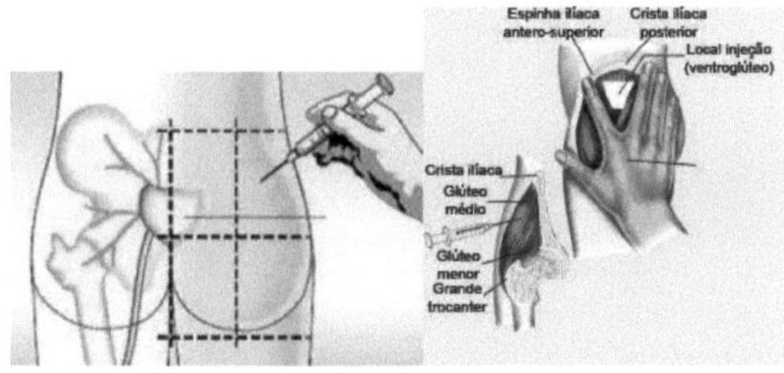

- Location: In the buttocks, divided into dorsogluteal (higher and lateral) and ventrogluteal (more anterior and lateral).
- Use: These muscles are suitable for larger volumes due to their greater muscle mass.
- Considerations: It is essential to avoid the sciatic nerve, especially in the dorsogluteal muscle, which requires precise technique to avoid injury.

3. **Quadriceps (rectus femoris and vastus lateralis):**

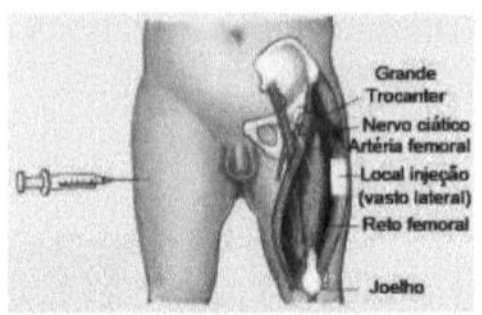

- Location: On the front of the thigh.
- Use: Also suitable for larger volumes and is a preferred option when access to the gluteal muscles is impractical.
- Advantages: Ease of access, especially for obese patients or young children, where other locations may be less accessible.

TABLE 2. Administration of intramuscular therapy: sites, volumes, positioning and anatomical landmarks (Ogston-Tuck, 2014)

Locations	Volume	Positioning	Anatomical references
Deltoid	Pre-school to school-age children : 0.5 to 1ml Teenagers and adults: 1-2ml	Standing or sitting, with your forearm on your abdomen to relax the syringe muscle	Identify the acromion. Locality 2 fingers or measure 2.5cm below this site and inject immediately below this site.
Ventrogluteal	Children from pre-school to school age: max. 2 ml Teenagers and adults 2.5-3ml	Lateral decubitus, with the nurse's back to the nurse with knee flexion or slight internal rotation of the foot for relaxation of the foot. muscle	Identify the greater trochanter and place the base of your hand on it (the nurse's right hand on the client's left hip or vice versa). Place your index finger on the iliac crest and spread your fingers so that A V. Inject into the centre of the V
Rectus femoris	Up to 5ml	Sitting or lying down, with the feet rotated slightly inwards to relax the muscles. muscle	Place the base of one hand on the greater trochanter and the base of the other hand on the knee, dividing the thigh into three parts. Administer to the anterior surface of the part upper middle third
Lateral vase	NB: max 1ml Latent: 1 to 2ml Adolescents: 1 to 2ml Adults: up to 5ml	Sitting or lying down, with the feet rotated slightly inwards to relax the muscles. muscle	Palpate the greater trochanter and knee joint; divide the distance between these two anatomical landmarks into thirds and use the middle third on the anterolateral surface of the thigh for injection.

Dorsogluteal	Teenagers and Adults: 1-4ml	Lying on Prone position	Visually divide the buttock into quadrants using an imaginary vertical and horizontal line and inject into the upper outer quadrant. Some authors suggest dividing this quadrant into another quadrant and using the Upper Outer Quadrant syringe in the upper outer quadrant.

The choice of the appropriate site for intramuscular injection depends not only on the amount of muscle tissue available, but also on the proximity of nerves and blood vessels. The injection technique must be meticulous to minimise the risk of complications such as pain, nerve damage or bruising. The training and experience of the healthcare professional are crucial to the safe performance of this procedure.

Here are the detailed steps for the safe preparation and administration of medicines by this route.

Preparation of Intramuscular Injectables

Preparing medicines for intramuscular administration involves several critical steps to ensure the safety and efficacy of the procedure:

1. **Hand hygiene:**
    - Hand hygiene is essential before preparing any medication to avoid contamination.
2. **Assessment of the patient's history:**
    - Know the patient's personal history and check for possible allergies to avoid adverse reactions.
3. **Checking the statute of limitations:**
    - Confirm the medicine to be administered, the prescribed dose, the route of administration and the planned date and time of administration.
4. **Confrontation with drugs:**
    - Compare the name and presentation of the medicine with the prescription and check the expiry date to ensure that the medicine is fit for use.

5. **Syringe and preparation of the medicine:**
    - Choose a suitable syringe, checking that the packaging is intact and within the expiry date.
    - Open the syringe packaging up to the end of the plunger and remove the syringe, ensuring that the plunger moves freely. Keep the tip of the syringe sterile.
    - Open the needle packaging at the coloured end and attach the needle firmly to the syringe. Release the needle guard without removing it and place the syringe in a sterile tray.
6. **Preparation of the solution:**
    - Inspect the solution to be injected to check that it is not cloudy or contains sediment, indicating possible contamination or instability. Open the ampoule carefully.
    - Hold the syringe and insert the needle into the solution, avoiding touching the bottom of the ampoule to avoid damaging the needle.
    - Aspirate the desired medication, tilting the ampoule as necessary to keep the needle submerged and prevent air from entering.
7. **Removing air from the syringe:**
    - Place the syringe upright, raise it to eye level to make it easier to see and expel the air by pushing the plunger until the solution appears at the tip of the needle.
8. **Reconstitution of medicines:**
    - For medicines that need to be reconstituted, make sure the powder is at the bottom of the bottle. Disinfect the rubber cap with an alcohol solution and let it dry before inserting the needle with the diluent.
    - Pour in the required volume of diluent, turn the bottle between your hands and shake gently until the powder is completely dissolved.
    - Inspect the solution to ensure there is no precipitation, insert the needle, invert the vial and aspirate the correct amount of the prepared solution.

Preparation for intramuscular injection

1. **Checking medication:**
    - Check out the 'right nine'

- make sure that the medicine is at the right temperature, especially if it is stored in the fridge.

2. **Choice of material:**
    - Use a syringe with adequate capacity for the prescribed dose and a needle of the right calibre and length to reach the muscle.
3. **Preparation of the injection site:**
    - The most common sites for IM injections include the deltoid muscle (upper arm), vastus lateralis (side of the thigh) and ventrogluteus (side of the hip).
    - Clean the area with an antiseptic solution and leave to dry naturally to reduce the risk of infection.

Medication Administration

4. **Administration Technician:**
    - Use a different needle for administration than for preparation, ensuring that the bevel is in perfect condition and that there is no residue that could cause pain. The drug should be administered at a rate of 1 ml per second, or as specified by the drug.
    - With clean, dry skin, relax the patient's muscle.
    - The recommended technique is similar to throwing a dart, which helps to minimise pressure and the accidental deposit of medication during needle insertion. The insertion angle should be 90 degrees to ensure that the drug is administered into the muscle.
    - Lightly aspirate the plunger to check that the needle is not in a blood vessel (if you see blood, remove the needle, change it and select another site).
        - Note: The World Health Organisation suggests that aspiration is only necessary in highly vascularised sites, such as the dorsogluteal muscle. However, recent studies indicate that aspiration may be unnecessary in clinical practice, except for this specific muscle.
    - Inject the medicine slowly and continuously.

Z-Injection Technique

Although less used among nurses in Portugal, the Z-injection technique is highly effective in preventing drug reflux:

- **Preparation:** Slide the skin and subcutaneous layers over the muscle layer using your index finger and thumb.
- **Needle insertion:** Hold the position and insert the needle in a single firm movement to penetrate the layers in the muscle.
- **Drug injection:** Administer the drug slowly, according to its characteristics.
- **Finish:** After waiting 10 seconds, apply a compress to the area, press lightly and remove the needle in one quick movement.
- **Post-injection care:** Avoid massaging the injection site to avoid dispersing the drug.

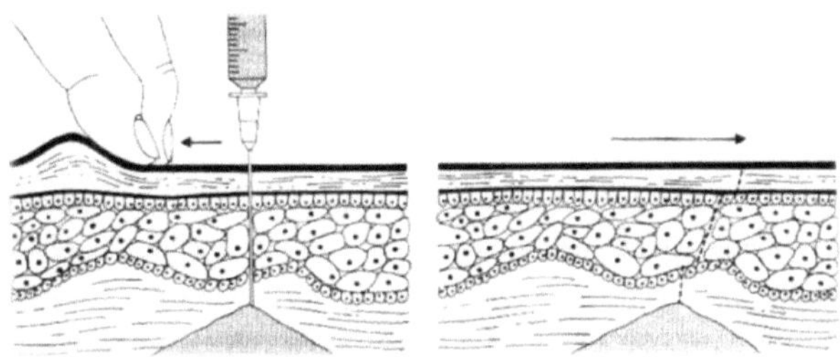

5. **After the injection:**
    - After administration, wait 10 seconds before removing the needle to prevent the drug from returning via the needle path. This step is omitted if the Z injection technique is used.
    - Apply pressure to the site with a sterile gauze pad to minimise bleeding.
    - Do not massage the injection site to avoid dispersing the drug outside the injection site and minimise discomfort.
6. **Safe Disposal:**
    - Dispose of needles and syringes in a sharps container.

Documentation and Monitoring

7. **Documentation:**

- Record all the details of the administration, including the date, time, injection site, medication, dose and any patient reaction.

8. **Patient monitoring:**
    - Observe the patient for any immediate adverse reactions.
    - Inform the patient about signs of infection or other complications at the injection site and when to seek medical attention.

Special considerations

- **Rotation of injection sites:**
    - It is important to rotate the injection sites to avoid the formation of scar tissue and to ensure consistent absorption of the drug.
- **Patient education:**
    - Explain to the patient the procedure and expectations after the injection, including care of the injection site and possible side effects.

The intramuscular administration of medicines is a common procedure that requires proper technique and specific knowledge to guarantee the safety and efficacy of the treatment. Following the correct steps and maintaining good hygiene practices are essential to prevent complications and promote the patient's well-being.

4.10. Administration of intravenous (IV) medication

Intravenous (IV) drug administration is a crucial method in healthcare that allows drugs to be introduced directly into the patient's bloodstream. This method is essential for treatments that require rapid and precise effects.

It involves injecting liquid substances directly into a vein using a needle or catheter. This method is one of the fastest for administering medicines and fluids into the circulatory system, allowing for almost immediate action.

Advantages of Administration IV

1. **Speed of action:** Allows an almost immediate response, which is vital in emergencies.

2. **Dosage accuracy:** The dosage can be precisely controlled, which is crucial for drugs that have narrow therapeutic windows.
3. **Continuous Administration:** Allows continuous infusion of medication or fluids, ideal for prolonged treatment.

Disadvantages of Administration IV

1. **Risks of infection: This** includes increased risks of infection, especially if asepsis is not strictly practised.
2. **Venous complications:** Can cause phlebitis, extravasation and thrombus formation.
3. **Immediate adverse reactions:** As the drug is administered directly into the bloodstream, adverse reactions can be faster and more severe.

Common venepuncture sites

1. **Forearm veins:** These include the basilic vein, cephalic vein and middle forearm veins, which are often used due to their easy accessibility and lower risk of complications.
2. **Arm**
3. **Antecubital region**

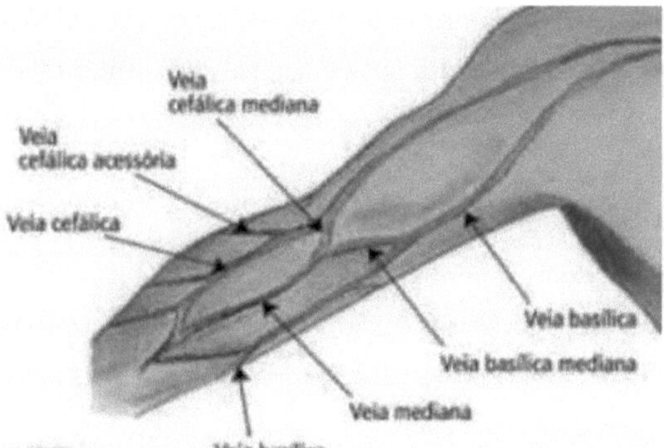

4. **Back of the hand**: Used especially in situations where other veins are less accessible, but present a greater risk of discomfort and complications.

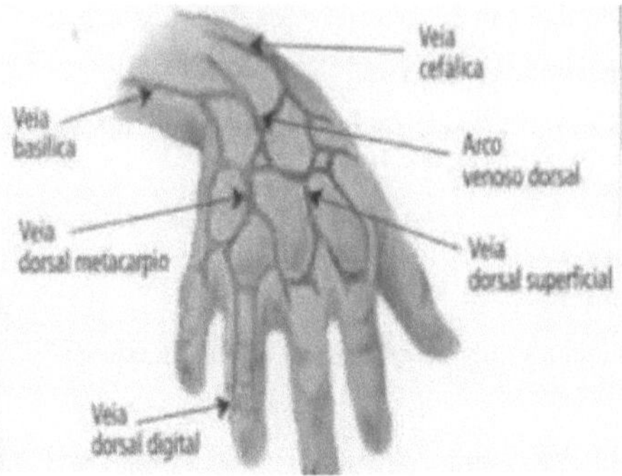

5. **Back of the foot: an** option in certain patients, such as in some paediatric cases, although it is less common due to a higher risk of infection.

Methods of administering IV medication

1. **Direct injection (Bolus):** Rapid administration of a single dose of medication directly into a vein, useful in emergency situations.
2. **Continuous Infusion:** Medication diluted in a bag of solution that is infused slowly, ideal for maintaining constant levels of the drug in the blood.
3. **Intermittent Infusion:** Administration of medication at regular intervals, usually through a venous access system that allows multiple doses without the need for multiple punctures.

Preparation for intravenous administration

1. **Prescription verification:**
    - Make sure that all the details on the prescription are correct, including the patient's name, the medicine, the dose, the route of administration and the planned time of administration.
2. **Hygienisation and material preparation:**
    - Wash your hands and wear gloves to prevent contamination.
    - Organise all the material needed for administration, such as syringes, needles, IV catheters, medicines and solutions for dilution, as required.
3. **Preparation of the medicine:**

- Inspect the medicine for colour and the presence of particles, and check the expiry date. Do not use the medicine if there are any changes.
- Prepare the medicine according to the manufacturer's instructions, ensuring correct dilution where applicable.

Drug Administration

4. **Choice of Insertion Site:**
    - Identify a suitable vein for inserting the IV catheter, preferably in the arm or hand. Avoid areas with damaged veins or signs of inflammation.
5. **Insertion of the IV catheter:**
    - Disinfect the chosen area with an antiseptic solution and allow it to dry completely.
    - Insert the catheter with aseptic technique, ensuring that the needle enters the vein at an appropriate angle. Confirm correct placement by observing venous return.
6. **Drug administration:**
    - Connect the syringe to the IV catheter and administer the drug in a controlled manner, adjusting the speed according to the drug's specifications.

Monitoring and Care After Administration

7. **Monitoring:**
    - Observe the patient closely during and after administration to identify signs of adverse reactions and inflammation, such as pain, oedema or redness at the injection site.
    - Ensure that the venous access remains clean and protected, using a sterile dressing if necessary.

Documentation and Patient Education

8. **Detailed documentation:**
    - Document all relevant information, including the date and time of administration, the insertion site, the type and quantity of medicine administered, as well as any observations on the patient's response.
9. **Patient education:**
    - Inform the patient about the procedure carried out, the expected effects of the medicine and any warning signs of possible complications.

Conclusion

On completing the study of this manual, nursing students will not only be equipped with in-depth technical knowledge of drug administration and therapeutic management, but also with a clear understanding of their vital role in promoting patient well-being and recovery. This manual serves as a robust foundation for future nurses to face the challenges of clinical practice, grounded in a perspective that values both technical competence and humanised care.

Virginia Henderson's philosophy, which emphasises the importance of assisting the individual so that they can carry out their own independent recovery as quickly as possible, is a cornerstone of this manual. According to Henderson, the essence of nursing practice lies in helping the individual, whether sick or healthy, to carry out the activities that contribute to their health or recovery (or to a peaceful death) that they would carry out unaided if they had the necessary strength, will or knowledge.

Incorporating Henderson's principles, this manual encourages nurses to adopt a holistic, patient-centred approach, where drug administration techniques are seen as an integral part of care that respects the patient's physical, emotional, social and spiritual needs. In doing so, we promote not only therapeutic efficacy, but also the dignity and independence of the patient, aligning care practices with the highest ethical principles.

By preparing nursing students to enter clinical practice with a solid foundation in technical skills and a rich understanding of patient-centred care, this manual serves as an essential resource that inspires nursing practice that is both technically and humanistically advanced. This resource is not only a guide to procedures and techniques, but also a source of inspiration for nurses who aspire to transform the lives of their patients, respecting their individuality and promoting recovery that transcends the physical to touch the psychological and emotional.

It is our hope that each reader of this handbook will not only acquire fundamental knowledge, but will also be inspired to follow Virginia Henderson's teachings, promoting a nursing practice that is deeply rooted in principles of compassionate and attentive care.

References

- Ana Fabíola Rebouças de, S., Queiroz, J. C. d., Vieira, A. N., Lilian Grace da Silva, S., & Érica Louise de Souza Fernandes, B. (2020). Medication errors and the risk factors associated with their prescription. *Enfermagem em foco.* https://doi.org/10.21675/2357-707x.2019.v10.n4.1900
- Azevedo, D. (2016) (Coord.) - The use of the subcutaneous approach in geriatrics and palliative care. An SBGG and ANCP guide for professionals. Rio de Janeiro: Brazilian Society of Geriatrics and Gerontology. Accessed on 28/02/2022. Available at https://sbgg.org.br//wp-content/uploads/2016/06/uso-da-via-subcutaneageriatria-cuidados-paliativos.pdf
- Balderrama, D. & Heering, H. (2018). Medication Administration: Intradermal Injection. Nursing practice & skill. Glendale, USA: Cinahl Information Systems.
- Camerini, F. G., Lage, J. S. L., Fassarella, C. S., & Franco, A. S. (2022). Evaluation of medication administration: identification of risks and implementation of safety barriers. *Journal of Nursing and Health.* https://doi.org/10.15210/jonah.v12i1.2248
- Caple, C. (2015). Medication Administration: Intradermal Injection. Nursing practice & skill. Glendale, USA: Cinahl Information Systems.
- Caple, C. & Heering, H. (2017). Medication Administration in Adults: Intramuscular. Nursing practice & skill. Glendale, USA: Cinahl Information Systems.
- Cinahl Information Systems (2017). Medication Administration in Adults: Intramuscular. Skills competency checklist. Glendale, USA: Cinahl Information Systems.
- Cinahl Information Systems (2017). Medication Administration in Paediatric Patients: Intramusucular. Skills competency checklist. Glendale, USA: Cinahl Information Systems.
- Cinahl Information Systems (2018). Medication Administration: Intradermal Injection. Skills competency checklist. Glendale, USA: Cinahl Information Systems.
- Cinahl Information Systems (2018). Medication Administration: Subcutaneous Injection. Skills competency checklist. Glendale, USA: Cinahl Information Systems.
- Diggle, J. (2015). Diabetes management and best practice in injection technique. Nurse Prescribing, 13(2), 72-78.
- Directorate-General for Health (2016). Standard 001/2016: Vaccination of children (under 6 years of age) belonging to tuberculosis risk groups with the BCG vaccine. Lisbon: Directorate-General for Health.
- Duque, F. A. T., Dias, E. F., Malta, J. S., Rodrigues, P. C., Lucas de Faria Martins, B., & Costa, J. M. d. (2022). Evaluation of paediatric prescription of hydroxyurea for patients with sickle cell disease. *O mundo da saúde.* https://doi.org/10.15343/0104-7809.202246369379i
- Felipe Lopes de Sousa, G., Lopes, N. M., Xavier, M. P., Sousa, S. F. d., Vale, B. N. d., & Santana, V. L. (2019). Elabora? Protocols for Administration. Oral solid medicines by nutritional tubes or Enteral. *Amazon Science & Health.* https://doi.org/10.18606/2318-1419/amazonia.sci.health.v7n1p26-49
- Figueredo, I. B., Fabiana Pinto de Almeida, B., & Nila Larisse Silva de, A. (2022). Types of errors in the preparation and administration of intravenous

medications: an integrative literature review. *Sustinere Journal.* https://doi.org/10.12957/sustinere.2021.55356

- Fontenele, N. Â. O., Vera Lúcia Mendes de Paula, P., Monteiro, A. R. M., Barros, L. M., & Rhanna Emanuela Fontenele Lima de, C. (2020). Clinical nursing care and patient safety in medication administration. *Research and Development Society.* https://doi.org/10.33448/rsd-v9i9.7052
- Freire, I. L. S., Lima, R. F. D., Santos, F. r. d., Silva, B., Medeiros, A. B. D., & George Felipe de Moura, B. (2020). Role of the nursing team in the preparation and administration of medications in a maternal intensive care unit. *Enfermagem Brasil.* https://doi.org/10.33233/eb.v19i2.1174
- Gelder, C. (2014). Good practice injection technique for children and young people with diabetes. children breastfeeding and young people,. 26 (7), 32-36.
- Greenway, K. (2014). Rituals in nursing: intramuscular injections. Journal of Clinical Nursing, 23, 3583 - 3588.
- Higa, C. M. L., Maria de Fátima Meinberg, C., Júnior, M. A. F., Flores, V. G. T., Andréia Insabralde de Queiroz, C., & Benites, P. T. (2021). Errors in drug administration through gastrointestinal catheters: an integrative review. *Health and Human Development.* https://doi.org/10.18316/sdh.v9i1.6463
- Hunter, J. (2008). Intramuscular injection techniques. Nursing Standard, 22(24), 35-40. 31
- Isabel Cristina da Silva, C., Oliveira, M. T. C., Silveira, C. P. C., & José Raul Rocha de Araújo, J. (2022). The increased risk of osteoporosis associated with chronic use of proton pump inhibitors: an integrative literature review. *Amazonian Journal of Pharmaceutical Sciences.* https://doi.org/10.17648/2675-5572.racf.v3n1.2
- Jaqueline Risolêta de Góis, C., Valle, K. R. d., Menezes, A. C., Santos, G. d., Schlosser, C. N., Edilene Aparecida Araújo da, S., Schlosser, T. C. M., & Trevisan, D. D. (2021). Simulation in teaching nurses to administer highly monitored drugs: a brief overview. *Research and Development Society.* https://doi.org/10.33448/rsd-v10i12.17576
- Jesus, M. C.; Trindade, C. S.; Lopes, J. & Ramos, A. L. (2020). Administration of intramuscular therapy in paediatrics: an integrative literature review. Ibero-American Journal of Health and Ageing. 6 April (1). 2117-2133.
- Kee, J.L., Hayes, E. R. & McCuistion L.E. (2012). Pharmacology: a nursing process approach. 7th ed., St. Louis: Elsevier Saunders.
- Ladebo, L., Foster, D. J. R., Abuhelwa, A. Y., Upton, R. N., Kongstad, K. T., Drewes, A. M., Christrup, L. L., & Olesen, A. E. (2019). Population pharmacokinetic-pharmacodynamic modelling of liquid and controlled-release formulations of oxycodone in healthy volunteers. *Basic Clinical Pharmacology or Toxicology.* https://doi.org/10.1111/bcpt.13330
- Laís Facioli Rosa Moreno da, C., Bonacim, C. A. G., Pereira, R. M. R., Gonella, J. M., Leclerc, J., & Gimenes, F. R. E. (2022). Programme to improve the quality of medication administration via nasal tube. *Ata Paulista de Enfermagem.* https://doi.org/10.37689/acta-ape/2022ao000934
- Lima, E. L. d., Valente, F. B. G., & Adenícia Custódia Silva e, S. (2022). Occurrence of errors in the preparation and administration of medication in an Emergency Care Unit. *Revista Eletrônica de Enfermagem.* https://doi.org/10.5216/ree.v24.68956
- Lima, M. E. F., Silva, L. T. D., Santo, A. d. E., Dias, W. L. R., Jéssyca Karolaine Carvalho da, S., Ana Beatriz Rodrigues Da, S., Millena Stephanie

Pereira Da, S., Lidiane Marinho da Silva, B., Oliveira, D. A. L., & Rosa Régia Sousa de, M. (2021). Nursing staff knowledge about safety in emergency medication administration / Nursing staff knowledge about emergency medication safety. *Revista Brasileira de Saúde Review.* https://doi.org/10.34119/bjhrv4n6-148

- Luana Carla Lima de, A., Tâmara Pimentel Gomes de, L., Fábio Palma Albarado da, S., & Quaresma, T. C. (2022). Laboratory and clinical analysis of treatment with direct-acting antiviral drugs in hepatitis C patients. *Research and Development Society.* https://doi.org/10.33448/rsd-v11i14.35756
- Lucas Soares da Nóbrega, S., Maria Vitória Ideão Leite da, R., & Batista, A. M. (2021). Prescription of medicines subject to special control in a municipality in the state of Seridó Potiguar, Brazil. *Infarma - Pharmaceutical Sciences.* https://doi.org/10.14450/2318-9312.v33.e2.a2021.pp167-174
- Maitê Lucas Alencar da, S., Souza, M. K. B., & Rosa Maria Ferreira de, A. (2019). Adverse drug events: analysis of data from a specialised hospital in the light of patient safety. *Scientific Knowledge.* https://doi.org/10.22614/resc-v8-n1-1108
- Mann, E. (2016). Injection (Intramuscular): Clinical Information. JBI.
- Manola, C. C. V., Evandro Bernardino Mendes de, M., Lau, Y. K. C., Bedin, L. P., Oliveira, M. V. d., Miriam Aparecida Inácio de, A., Magda Ribeiro de Castro, S., & Machado, P. S. (2020). Knowing, from the puerperal woman's perspective, the relevance of the childbirth care project based on Virginia Henderson's theory. *Enfermagem (São Paulo).* https://doi.org/10.36489/nursing.2020v23i265p4181-4192
- Mardem Augusto Paiva Rocha, J., Francisco Lucas de Lima, F., Pinho, L. F., Santos, S. L. d., Ilana Maria Brasil do Espírito, S., Bruna Furtado Sena de, Q., Oliveira, M. C. d., Freitas, E. P., Ayla Cristina Rodrigues Ramos da, C., Francisca Jéssica Abreu da, S., Rodrigues, M. I. R., Karine do Nascimento Miranda Martins, G., Brenda Lícia Martins da, S., Jadson de Farias de Farias, S., & Araújo, L. V. (2019). Challenges and perspectives for the safe administration of medicines by nursing. *Coleção Saúde da Revista Eletrônica.* https://doi.org/10.25248/reas.e452.2019
- Maria Regina Tavares dos, S., Ana Paula Rocha de, L., & Silva, R. C. (2021). Potential drug-nutrient interactions in institutionalised elderly in Campo Mourão-PR. *Wise Men - Journal of Health and Biology.* https://doi.org/10.54372/sb.2021.v16.2919
- Maria Valdênia Lima do, Ó., & Siqueira, L. d. P. (2021). The importance of pharmaceutical assistance in drug-related problems: an integrative review. *Research and Development Society.* https://doi.org/10.33448/rsd-v10i15.22662
- Mauro, E. A. C., & Carreiro, M. d. A. (2019). Errors and violations in the preparation and administration of medications in the intensive care unit. *Revista Pró-Universus* https://doi.org/10.21727/rpu.v10i1.1637
- Meneses, K. S., Costa, R. S. N., Silva-Barbosa, C. E. d., Cunha, L. N., Moraes, J. J. d., Brito, L. S. B., Reis, D. F., Almeida, C. G. d., Brandão, P. P., Xavier, M. d. S., Fabíola Pessôa Figueira de, S., Bethoven, H. B., Nunes, C., Sousa, C. M. d., & Evangelista, B. F. (2023). Strategies for the prevention of adverse events in the administration of medicines by the nursing team. *Research and Development Society.* https://doi.org/10.33448/rsd-v12i1.38964
- Neto, I.G. (2008). Use of the subcutaneous route in clinical practice. Society of Internal Medicine, 15(4). 277-283

- Ogston-Tuck, S. (2014) Subcutaneous injection technique: an evidence-based approach. Nursing Standard 29(3), 53-58.
- Ogston-Tuck, S. (2014). Intramuscular injection technique: an evidence-based approach. Nursing Standard, 29(4), 52-59.
- Peregrino, J. & Schub, E. (2017). Medication Administration in Children: Subcutaneous Injection. Nursing practice & skill. Glendale, USA: Cinahl Information Systems.
- Pinheiro, T. S., Mendonça, E. T. d., Siman, A. G., Carvalho, C. A. d., Zanelli, F. P., & Marilane de Oliveira Fani, A. (2021). Medication administration in an emergency department: actions taken and challenges for safe practices. *Enfermagem em foco.* https://doi.org/10.21675/2357-707x.2020.v11.n3.3172
- Raharja, M. L. T., Rista, R., Kholif, S. N., Rohyani, Y., Prasetyo, B., & Santoso, A. P. A. (2022). Comparison of Virginia Henderson's Theory with Abraham Maslow's Theory of Basic Human Concepts. *Journal of Complementarity in Health.* https://doi.org/10.36086/jch.v2i2.1499
- Sandra, R. M. d. O., Oliveira, P. P., Rosa, L. S., Alves, J. D. S., Quézia Louize Da Costa de, A., & Brito, T. (2020). Enteral drug administration: nursing knowledge and praxis regarding therapeutic response. *Enfermagem (São Paulo).* https://doi.org/10.36489/nursing.2020v23i264p4048-4071
- Santos, R. C., Goulart, A. C., Lotufo, P. A., & Santos, I. S. (2020). Frequency and reasons for non-administration and discontinuation of medications during an acute coronary syndrome event. ERICO study. *Brazilian Archive of Cardiology.* https://doi.org/10.36660/abc.20190317
- Schub, T. and C. Caple (2015). Medication Administration in Adults: Intramuscular. D. Pravikoff, Editor, EBSCO Publishing: Ipswich, Massachusetts.
- Siboni, F. H., Behboudi, F., Mohebbi, K., Majidi, S., Yaghobi, Y., & Carroll, K. (2023). Virginia Henderson's writings on the nature of nursing: an example of nursing practice. *Nursing Science Quarterly.* https://doi.org/10.1177/08943184221150255
- Silva, A. O. d., Barbosa, A. A., Ana Paula de Souza, C., Rolim, I. A. A., Santos, R. F. d., Borges, J. M. P., & Lemos, G. d. S. (2021). Potential drug-alcohol interactions in alcoholic patients attended by an Alcohol and Drug Psychosocial Care Centre. *Research and Development Society.* https://doi.org/10.33448/rsd-v10i9.17697
- Sisson, H. (2015). Aspiration during the intramuscular injection procedure: a systematic literature review. Journal of Clinical Nursing, 24, 2368 - 2375.
- Stelman Teixeira Moreira dos, S. (2021). Factors associated with the occurrence of errors in the preparation and administration of intravenous medications: a systematic review of the literature. *Annals of Scientific Initiation Seminars.* https://doi.org/10.13102/semic.vi24.7183
- Teixeira, L. d. S., Souza, D. R., Fantin, A. B., & Christian Diniz Lima e, S. (2021). Interactions of allopathic medicines with herbal medicines based on ginkgo biloba and valeriana officinalis. *Research and Development Society.* https://doi.org/10.33448/rsd-v10i12.20444
- Torres, P. C., Fonseca, L. B., Cândido, R. F., Joyce Costa Melgaço de, F., & Pádua, C. M. d. (2021). Experiences of users of a drug information centre about the work of professional pharmacists. *Brazilian Journal of Hospital Pharmacy and Health Services.* https://doi.org/10.30968/rbfhss.2021.123.0617
- Walsh, K. and C. Caple (2015). Medication Administration in Neonates: Intramuscular. D. Pravikoff, Editor, EBSCO Publishing: Ipswich, Massachusetts.

- Walsh, K. and T. Schub (2017). Medication Administration in Paediatric Patients: Intramuscular. Nursing practice & skill. Glendale, USA: Cinahl Information Systems
- Zamboni, W. C. (2023). Effect of obesity on the pharmacokinetics and pharmacodynamics of anticancer agents. *Journal of Clinical Pharmacology.* https://doi.org/10.1002/jcph.2326

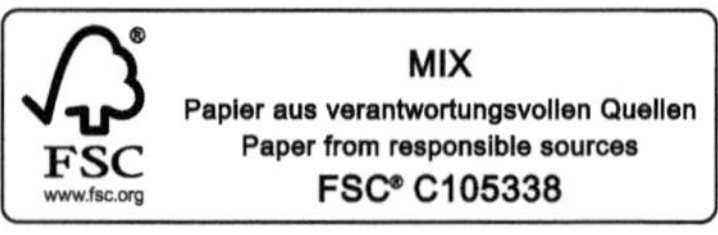

Printed by Books on Demand GmbH, Norderstedt / Germany